SCOPE and STANDARDS
of
Pediatric Oncology
Nursing Practice

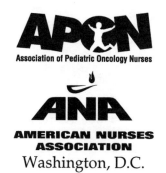

Association of Pediatric Oncology Nurses

AMERICAN NURSES
ASSOCIATION
Washington, D.C.

Library of Congress Cataloging-in-Publication Data

Scope and standards of pediatric oncology nursing practice / Association
   of Pediatric Oncology Nurses, American Nurses Association.
        p. cm.
      Includes bibliographical references.
        1. Tumors in children—Nursing. I. Association of Pediatric
   Oncology Nurses (U.S.)
   RC281.C4 S386 2000
   610.73′62—dc21   00-048523

Published by
American Nurses Publishing
600 Maryland Avenue
Suite 100 West
Washington, DC 20024-2571

ISBN 1-55810-154-3

PONP20   2M   11/00

ACKNOWLEDGMENTS

Authors

Jill Brace O'Neill, RN-CS, MS, PNP, CPON
APON Practice Committee Chair
Coordinator of Clinical Research
Boston Children's Hospital, Boston, Massachusetts

Mary Jo Cleaveland, RN, MS
Clinical Nurse Specialist
The Children's Hospital, Denver, Colorado

Kathy Forte, RN, MS, CPNP
APON Scope of Practice Task Force Chair
Advanced Practice Nurse, AFLAC Cancer Center
Children's Health Care of Atlanta, Atlanta, Georgia

Jeanne Harvey, RN, MSN, CS, PNP, CPON
Pediatric Nurse Practitioner, David B. Perini Jr. Quality of Life Clinic
Dana-Farber Cancer Institute, Boston, Massachusetts

Casey Hooke, RN, MSN, CPON
Clinical Nurse Specialist, Pediatric Hematology/Oncology
Children's Hospitals and Clinics, Minneapolis, Minnesota

Katherine Patterson Kelly, RN, MN, CPON
Clinical Nurse Specialist
Children's Hospital at University of Missouri Hospitals and
    Clinics, Columbia, Missouri

Revonda Mosher, RN, MSN, CPNP, CPON
Advanced Practice Clinician, Hematology/Oncology
Children's National Medical Center, Washington, DC
Mary Baron Nelson, RN, MS, CPNP, CPON
Nurse Practitioner, LIFE Program
Children's Hospital, Los Angeles, California

Theresa Dunn Sievers, RN, MS
Director of Pediatric Oncology Nursing
Dana-Farber Cancer Institute, Boston, Massachusetts

Reviewers

Alice Ettinger, RN, MSN, CPNP, CPON
Program Coordinator, Division of Pediatric Hematology-Oncology
Saint Peter's University Hospital, New Brunswick, New Jersey

Donna Betcher, RN, MSN, CPNP
Pediatric Nurse Practitioner, Pediatric Oncology
Mayo Clinic, Rochester, Minnesota

Georgina Bru, RN, MA
Director, Children's Hospital at Dartmouth
Dartmouth-Hitchock Medical Center, Lebanon, New Hampshire

Janet A. Deatrick, RN, PhD, FAAN
Task Force Chair, Statement of the Scope and Standards of
    Advanced Practice Nursing,
The Society of Pediatric Nurses
Associate Professor, University of Pennsylvania School of
    Nursing, Philadelphia, Pennsylvania

Debra Eshelman, RN, MSN, CPNP
Advanced Practice Nurse, After the Cancer Experience Program
Children's Medical Center of Dallas, Dallas, Texas

Ria Hawks, RN, MS, CPON
Clinical Nurse Specialist, Pediatric Oncology
Babies and Children's Hospital of New York, New York,
    New York

Nancy Noonan, RN, MS
Clinical Nurse Specialist
Children's Hospital, Oakland, California

Janis Ryan Murray, RN, MSN, PNP, CPON
Pediatric Nurse Practitioner, Division of
    Pediatric Hematology-Oncology
Duke University Medical Center, Durham, North Carolina

Angela Toles, RN, BSN
Staff nurse, Ambulatory Care Unit
St. Jude Children's Research Hospital, Memphis, Tennessee

Leslie Wagner-McMahon, RN, MSN
Health Care Consultant
Palm Harbor, Florida

We recognize the following individuals who participated in the
development and review of APON's 1987 *Scope of Practice and
Outcome Standards of Practice for Pediatric Oncology Nursing*:

Georgina Bru, RN, MA, CAN
Joan Chiavello RN, MS
Genevieve Foley, RN, MSN
Karen Hegranes, RN, MS
Carolyn Walker, RN, PhD
Linda Wofford, RN, MSN, PNP-C
Penelope Wright, RN, MS

CONTENTS

PREFACE

A specialty nursing organization is responsible for establishing, maintaining, and revising standards of nursing care that are relevant to the population these nurses serve. For the Association of Pediatric Oncology Nurses (APON), children and adolescents with cancer and their families are the focus of nursing care. For the purpose of this document, the word "child" is used to describe any child or adolescent, from birth to 21 years of age. When the word adolescent is specifically used, it is meant to include children from 12 to 21 years of age.

In 1978, the APON developed Standards of Nursing Practice for the pediatric oncology nurse, which were revised in 1987 to reflect both nursing process and outcome standards, including statements on the Scope of Practice (Bru et al. 1987). The changing healthcare environment has prompted the latest revision: *Scope of Practice and Outcome Standard of Practice for Pediatric Oncology Nurses* (APON 2000) incorporates key aspects from the *Code for Nurses with Interpretive Statements* (ANA 1985) and previously published standards from organizations such as the American Nurses Association (ANA 1998, 1996), the Society of Pediatric Nursing (Deatrik et al. 1998; Bartolone et al. 1996), and the Oncology Nursing Society (Lester, Glass, and Owen 1997; Ryan et al. 1996). This document was developed in accordance with ANA 2000.

This document provides

- statements concerning competence for basic and advanced clinical pediatric oncology nursing practice.

- a definition of pediatric oncology nursing and a description of the expected outcomes for the child and family.

- guidelines for nurses, other health care providers, payers, consumers, and policy makers in evaluating the effectiveness, quality, and appropriateness of health care services for the child with cancer.

SCOPE OF PEDIATRIC ONCOLOGY NURSING PRACTICE

History of Pediatric Oncology Nursing

In the early 1960s, children diagnosed with cancer began to have sustained remissions, with some even being considered cured. With more children with cancer living longer, pediatric nurses in greater numbers began to specialize in the care of these children. In the mid 1970s, pediatric oncology nursing emerged as a subspecialty within pediatric nursing. The nurses' role was to administer chemotherapy, provide patient and family education, and care for children at the end of life.

The formal organization of specialty nursing practice and the development of advanced practice nursing roles in pediatric oncology facilitated the development of pediatric oncology as a subspecialty. In 1973, the first gathering of pediatric oncology nurses was held at the national conference of the Association for the Care of Children's Health. The following year marked the founding of APON, which incorporated in 1976. Certification for pediatric oncology nurses (CPON) became available in 1993.

Contemporary Issues and Trends

The Association of Pediatric Oncology Nurses recognizes the complex needs of children diagnosed with cancer and their families. Issues related to the care of the child and family remain the central focus of the association's activities. Several important contemporary issues in society and in the delivery of health care have impacted nursing care of children and families. Significant changes have included advances in technology and science, the increasing numbers of survivors of childhood cancer, the impact of cooperative group clinical trials, and the shift of care to the ambulatory setting and the subsequent burden that this places on the family.

Technological and pharmacologic advances made in the past decade have improved the tools used to diagnose and treat childhood cancers. Current treatment regimens are intensive and complex, lasting from months to years, and involve multiple treatment modalities. In addition, improved supportive care has allowed patients to tolerate the increasing intensity of treatment regimens.

Because of these advances, it is estimated that 1 in 900 people ages 15 to 45 years of age will be a survivor of childhood cancer. The increasing number of childhood cancer survivors over the past decade has brought to light the special needs and issues they must face. Pediatric oncology nurses have an important role in the care of survivors. This role includes monitoring, assessing, and treating children and adult survivors for the effects of treatment that emerge long after the completion of therapy, as well as teaching survivors about healthy lifestyles and how to minimize the late effects for which they may be at risk.

The increase in cure rate of children with cancer is in part due to the impact of cooperative group clinical trials. Most children diagnosed with cancer are enrolled in a clinical trial at a comprehensive cancer center. Advances are made as large numbers of children are enrolled in clinical trials, such as improved survival, reduction of treatment- related complications/toxicities and improvement in overall quality of life. Recent studies have reported that adolescents have not been afforded the same opportunity to enroll in clinical trials (Bleyer et al. 1997). Pediatric oncology nurses have a role in educating and advocating for adolescent patients and their families regarding clinical trials.

The health care system in the United States has undergone significant changes with the introduction of prospective payment systems and diagnosis related groups (DRGs). There has also been an increase in the number of health maintenance organizations, and a reduction in the number of those insured. Care is delivered in complex hospital and health care systems. In an effort to reduce costs and maintain normalcy for the family, the site of pediatric oncology care has shifted from the hospital environment to outpatient and home care settings. Coupled with the increasing intensity and complexity of care, the burden of care has increased for the child and family. To provide care for their children, parents and families require more information and education related to disease and treatment.

Adaptation to the ambulatory care environment means normalizing life as much as possible for children and families. Because school plays such an important role in the lives of children, facilitating a return to school for academic achievement and continued development of social skills is important. Pediatric oncology nurses must advocate for the child in the school environment and encourage participation in this normalizing activity by promoting school re-entry and hospital-based tutorial programs.

The pediatric oncology nurse must understand the impact of the cancer experience on the child and family and recognize how to incorporate this into the plan of care. Knowledge of the available community resources and close working relationships with these resources is vital in advocating for the rights and needs of children with cancer. Over the past decade, there have been changes in the nuclear family unit, the development of a greater appreciation for different cultures, and an increase in the financial burden placed on families related to health care. The pediatric oncology nurse must be aware of the economic factors that hamper access to care.

All of these changes in society and health care delivery systems have changed the role of the pediatric oncology nurse and created new challenges to delivering expert, evidenced- based nursing care. The increased intensity and complexity of cancer care and the shift of care to the ambulatory care setting requires more intensive monitoring, coordination of services across all sites of care, and ongoing communication between the child, family, and the health care team. Pediatric oncology nurses are in a key position to continually measure and improve the outcomes of pediatric oncology nursing care.

Description of Pediatric Oncology Nursing

Pediatric oncology nursing is defined as the nursing care of children with cancer and their families in a variety of health care settings. Both the clinical nurse and the advanced practice nurse (APN) practice in diverse settings, which may include the hospital, ambulatory clinic, hospice, physician's office, school or other community setting, and home. Pediatric oncology nursing blends the expert practices of pediatrics and oncology nursing care. Pediatric oncology nursing requires a comprehensive understanding of the growth and development of children within the context of the family as well as the social and cultural environments in which they live. In addition, knowledge of cancer, cancer treatment, supportive care, and subsequent psychosocial issues is essential.

The organizing framework for the standards of care lays the groundwork for both the clinical nurse and the advanced practice nurse. This framework includes seven different areas, which include physical care, growth and development, psychosocial care, education, palliative care, long-term survival, and prevention and early detection. Specific interventions for each of these categories are outlined in the standards of care. It is the expectation that the clinical nurse and the advanced practice nurse focus on one or more of these seven areas as appropriate.

Pediatric oncology nursing practice is dedicated to providing expert, evidence-based nursing care for children with cancer and their families. The role of the pediatric oncology nurse includes direct patient care, education, advocacy, consultation, research, and management of health care delivery systems (APON 1995).

The clinical nurse and the advanced practice nurse are expected to be lifetime learners. This may be accomplished by attending conferences, obtaining continuing education credits, and pursuing other educational opportunities as appropriate (Hockenberry-Eaton 1998). Certification in pediatric oncology nursing is available for the clinical nurse. There is currently no certification available for the advanced practice nurse that is specific to pediatric oncology. However, advanced practice nurses may pursue certification in primary care, advanced oncology nursing, or in other areas as appropriate.

Pediatric Oncology Clinical Nurse

The pediatric oncology clinical nurse is a licensed registered nurse (RN) who demonstrates clinical knowledge and skill in the subspecialty of pediatric oncology nursing. Pediatric oncology nurses are responsible for adhering to pediatric oncology nursing standards as designated in this document, *Scope and Standards of Pediatric Oncology Nursing Practice*.

Pediatric Oncology Advanced Practice Nurse

Although the advanced practice registered nurse (APRN) title is commonly identified and referenced in the nursing literature and other nursing specialties, the pediatric oncology advanced practice nurse (APN) is the most frequently used term in this specialty describing a licensed, registered nurse prepared with a minimum of a master's degree, who has acquired advanced knowledge in pediatric oncology nursing. The pediatric oncology advanced practice nurse must demonstrate competencies in all areas of basic practice in addition to the APN standards. The advanced practice nurse may function as a clinical nurse, clinical nurse specialist, nurse practitioner, or in a combined or blended role. Specific state regulations may limit certain practices or procedures, such as prescriptive privileges. The inclusive title of APN has emerged in response to the need for uniform titles within the nursing profession. APON recognizes this blended title in documents and publications except when specific role functions are being described.

STANDARDS OF PEDIATRIC ONCOLOGY
CLINICAL NURSING PRACTICE

Role of Standards

Standards of care and professional performance describe the roles and responsibilities of the pediatric oncology nurse. The standards of care may be applied in all settings and across the continuum of care, including physical care, growth and development, psychosocial care, education, palliative care, long-term survival, and prevention/early detection.

Standards of Care

Standards of care pertain to professional nursing activities demonstrated by the nurse through the nursing process. This process includes assessment, diagnosis, outcome identification, planning, implementation, and evaluation.

Standards of Professional Performance

Standards of professional performance reflect the expectations for professional behavior, including activities related to quality of care, performance appraisal, education, collegiality, ethics, collaboration, research, and resource utilization.

STANDARDS OF CARE:
PEDIATRIC ONCOLOGY CLINICAL NURSE

Standard I. Assessment

The pediatric oncology nurse collects and documents data regarding the child and family.

Rationale

Assessment of the child's physical and psychosocial needs leads to the development of an appropriate plan of care for the child and family.

Measurement Criteria

The pediatric oncology nurse:

- A. Systematically collects data that is pertinent to the needs of the child and family.
- B. Collects data from the child, family and friends, and other health care providers.
- C. Collects data using appropriate assessment techniques and instruments.
- D. Collects data in the following areas as appropriate, through assessment of:
    1. Physical care, which may include:
        a. Symptoms by systems.
        b. Physical status of vital functions by assessing vital signs, laboratory data, general appearance, nutrition, and behavior.
        c. Parent's comfort level with assisting with or providing physical care for the child.
        d   Knowledge of common childhood illnesses and their management in the child with cancer.
        e. Knowledge of well-child health maintenance issues that may be different in the child with cancer.

f.   Methods of symptom and/or pain management and complementary therapies.

g.   Alterations in protective mechanisms, mobility, elimination, ventilation, circulation or comfort.

2. Growth and development, which may include:

a.   Current stage of growth and development by using assessment tools, developmental milestones, growth chart, and child/parent history.

b.   Level of interaction between child and parent(s).

c.   Impact of disease and treatment on the child's developmental level and tasks.

d.   Child's level of success in interpersonal relationships.

e.   Child and family's coping strategies and level of adjustment.

f.   Parents' ability to allow child to be independent appropriate to developmental level.

g.   Effects of body image changes on the child's developing self-concept.

h.   Impact of diseases and treatment on school attendance, academic achievement, and peer interaction.

3. Psychosocial care, which may include:

At time of diagnosis:

a.   Structure and roles of family, family interactions, lifestyle, and communication styles.

b.   Educational/occupational/life experiences that impact perception and understanding of cancer diagnosis.

c.   Cultural and spiritual traditions.

d.   Emotional responses to diagnosis (shock, disbelief, anger, grief, guilt).

e.   Effectiveness of support systems available to family.

f.   Factors that place the family at high risk for difficulty in coping.

g. Need for referral to financial resources/information.

During treatment:

a. Family adjustment to caring for the child with cancer across settings and adaptation to burden of care.

b. Impact on family dynamics (marriage, employment, finances).

c. Family and child's adaptation to school re-entry or home- bound instruction.

d. Sibling adaptation to new lifestyle.

e. Family adherence to cancer treatment plan.

At end of treatment:

a. Response to end of therapy and change in frequency of clinic visits.

b. Re-integration to life without cancer treatment.

c. Fear/anxiety about completion of treatment.

d. Potential psychosocial long-term effects of cancer (post-traumatic stress, risk-taking behavior, isolation).

At relapse:

a. Emotional responses to relapse.

b. Family history of response to crisis and adaptation skills.

c. Family support systems and their ability to sustain support.

4. Education, which may include:

a. Developmental and cognitive level of the child.

b. Child and family's knowledge of the diagnostic tests, diagnosis, prognosis, treatment, side effects, symptom management, and care at home.

c. Family's readiness to learn and preferred method of learning.

d. Formal and informal education/literacy level.

    e.   Availability of resources for non-English speaking families.

    f.   Availability of community, clinic, and home resources to continue the teaching process.

5. Palliative care, which may include:

    a.   Child's/family's understanding of the dying process and the goals of care.

    b.   Child's level of comfort.

    c.   Interventions that alleviate pain and promote comfort.

    d.   Support systems in the family and community.

    e.   Ability of caregiver to provide care to the child in the home or other setting.

    f.   Impact of prognosis on the siblings.

    g.   Understanding of child's/family's desires regarding end of life care.

6. Long-term survival, which may include:

    a.   Understanding of potential late effects of treatment based on treatment received.

    b.   Understanding of the plan for follow-up care after active treatment ends.

    c.   Coping style of the child and family and ability to transition to the "survivor" role.

    d.   Understanding of the availability of survivor clinics and/or transition clinics for adult survivors.

7. Prevention and early detection, which may include:

    a.   Identification of risk factors for second cancers.

    b.   Knowledge of warning signs and symptoms of cancer.

    c.   Understanding of healthy lifestyle behaviors especially regarding diet, exercise, cancer prevention, and cancer screening.

E. Documents data in the medical record.

Standard II. Diagnosis

The pediatric oncology nurse uses assessment data from nursing and other disciplines to determine diagnoses.

Rationale

Diagnoses help the pediatric oncology nurse to identify problems and to subsequently determine appropriate interventions, including the expected outcomes, the plan, and the evaluation.

Measurement Criteria

The pediatric oncology nurse:

A. Determines actual or potential diagnoses from assessment data.

B. Develops diagnoses that are age and developmentally appropriate, and culturally relevant.

C. Ensures that the diagnoses address physical care, growth and development, psychosocial care, palliative care, long-term survival, and prevention and early detection, as appropriate.

D. Communicates with the child and family and other members of the health care team to validate and prioritize the diagnoses.

E. Documents the diagnoses in the child's medical record to facilitate the determination of expected outcomes and plan of care.

Standard III. Outcome Identification

The pediatric oncology nurse identifies expected outcomes specific to the child and family.

Rationale

The identification of expected outcomes allows the pediatric oncology nurse to work with the child and family to meet the mutual goals of care. The expected outcomes include adequate education,

11

optimal growth and development, optimal physical and emotional health, prevention of toxicity, early detection of potential second malignancies, limited late effects, or a comfortable death.

Measurement Criteria

The pediatric oncology nurse:

A. Derives expected outcomes from diagnoses.

B. Designs outcomes that are mutually formulated with the child, family, and other health care team members as appropriate.

C. Ensures that outcomes are age and developmentally appropriate and culturally relevant.

D. Designs time-specific, realistic, and measurable outcomes.

E. Formulates outcomes that are congruent with the existing treatment plan.

F. Develops outcomes in the following areas as appropriate, but not limited to:

 1. Physical care, which may include:

    The child/family:

    a. Demonstrates proficiency in performing necessary physical and emotional care, including teaching and promoting self- care behaviors.

    b. Communicates appropriate interventions for common childhood illnesses.

    c. Verbalizes understanding of well child health maintenance, including what may be different in a child with cancer.

    d. Identifies appropriate methods of symptom or pain management.

    e. Describes appropriate interventions for real or potential alterations in protective mechanisms, mobility, elimination, ventilation, circulation, or comfort.

2. Growth and development, which may include:

The child:

   a. Demonstrates mastery and overcomes fears related to disease and treatment.

   b. Demonstrates independence appropriate to developmental level.

   c. Participates in daily care/engages in self-care as appropriate to developmental level.

   d. Maintains normalcy in life as much as possible through parental involvement, structure, and flexibility from caregivers, continued relationships with peers, school re- entry/tutoring, age-appropriate play/social activities, age- appropriate physical activities.

   e. Maintains growth patterns as plotted on the growth chart.

   f. Demonstrates mastery of language, social, and motor skills appropriate to developmental level.

The parent(s):

   a. Maintains discipline and consistency in approach to parenting; continues to have appropriate expectations of child.

   b. Establishes a routine appropriate to child's developmental level.

   c. Supports child's autonomy in learning about disease and treatment.

   d. Verbalizes understanding of cancer's impact on child's growth and development and assesses success of interventions to manage delays.

3. Psychosocial care, which may include:

At time of diagnosis, the family:

   a. Identifies and expresses emotions consistent with cultural background.

   b. Describes plan of care for child while hospitalized and at home.

13

c. Develops plan for addressing financial issues.

d. Explains diagnosis and treatment to the child and siblings as appropriate.

e. Demonstrates ability to participate in care.

During treatment, the family:

a. Verbalizes acceptance of diagnosis.

b. Verbalizes understanding of treatment plan and demonstrates compliance.

c. Utilizes available support systems (extended family, friends, spiritual/cultural community).

d. Establishes new "normal" in family routines and lifestyle.

e. Demonstrates ability to provide emotional support to child.

f. Demonstrates ability to provide support to siblings by inclusion in treatment routines and spending individual time with each child.

At end of treatment, the family:

a. Identifies and verbalizes feelings about completing therapy.

b. Adapts to treatment discontinuation by asking questions and verbalizing concerns.

c. Recognizes child's unique needs for follow-up care.

At relapse, the family:

a. Identifies and expresses emotions consistent with cultural background.

b. Verbalizes understanding of impact of relapse.

c. Participates in decision-making regarding treatment options.

4. Education, which may include:

The child/family:

a. Verbalize understanding of disease, treatment options, and potential side effects.

b. Demonstrate understanding of treatment by complying with recommended home care practices.

c. Share in the ongoing decision-making process as developmentally and culturally appropriate.

d. Identify resources for continued learning and support.

5. Palliative care, which may include:

The child/family:

a. Share in decision-making regarding end of life choices.

b. Communicate changes in comfort level or physical condition that will impact the child's well-being.

c. Acknowledge how to contact health care provider if symptoms worsen or level of comfort is not optimal.

d. Identify personal, professional, and spiritual resources that will assist the family in coping with the process of dying and bereavement.

6. Long-term survival, which may include:

The survivor/family:

a. Describe cancer treatment received, including chemotherapeutic agents, radiation sites, and surgeries.

b. Describe actual/potential late effects from the treatment received and understands follow-up plans for screening and health maintenance.

c. Verbalize understanding of long-term follow-up for prevention, monitoring, and early treatment of real or potential late effects of cancer treatment.

d. Utilize community, academic, and medical resources to achieve maximum quality of life after cancer.

7. Prevention and early detection, which may include:

The child/family:

a. Describe healthy lifestyle behaviors that will decrease chances of developing a secondary malignancy or other illness.

b. Describe cancer warning signs.

c. Identify risk factors for the development of cancer.

d. Describe cancer therapy that may increase risk of developing a secondary malignancy.

Standard IV. Planning

The pediatric oncology nurse develops an individualized plan that prescribes interventions to attain expected outcomes.

Rationale

A comprehensive and individualized care plan guides the health care team in implementing interventions that facilitate the achievement of expected outcomes.

Measurement Criteria

The pediatric oncology nurse:

A. Bases the plan of care on current knowledge of pediatric and oncologic nursing care.

B. Considers the age and cognitive ability of the child in formulating the plan of care.

C. Includes the patient and family in the development of the plan of care.

D. Considers the social, financial, spiritual, and cultural aspects of the family.

E. Includes physical and psychosocial interventions.

F. Includes a plan for education of the patient and family.

G. Creates a plan that provides for continuity of care.

H. Collaborates to develop and establish priorities for the plan of care with health care team members.

I. Documents the plan of care in the medical record.

Standard V. Implementation

The pediatric oncology nurse implements the plan of care to achieve the expected outcomes of the child and family.

Rationale

Implementation of the plan of care is designed to prevent or treat health care problems associated with the diagnosis of cancer. The overall goal is to improve the child's health status, promote quality of life, and facilitate optimal family functioning.

Measurement Criteria

The pediatric oncology nurse:

  A. Collaborates with other members of the health care team to implement interventions that are outlined in the plan of care.

  B. Coordinates delivery of care across health care settings.

  C. Participates in clinical trials by understanding and following the protocol for each patient, and explaining the rationale and schedule to the family.

  D. Ensures that the interventions are safe, timely, appropriate, and implemented in a caring manner.

  E. Ensures that interventions are age appropriate.

  F. Adjusts interventions to meet the needs of the child and family.

  G. Includes the child and family in the implementation process.

  H. Documents interventions in the medical record.

Standard VI. Evaluation

The pediatric oncology nurse evaluates the child and family's progress toward attainment of the expected outcomes.

Rationale

The plan of care and the impact of the interventions are continually evaluated and subsequently changed to meet the needs of the child and family and attain expected outcomes.

Measurement Criteria

The pediatric oncology nurse:

A. Collects data pertaining to the child and family's response to interventions.

B. Includes the patient, family, and other members of the health care team in the evaluation process when appropriate.

C. Utilizes an evaluation process that is systematic, ongoing, and criterion based.

D. Compares actual findings to expected outcomes.

E. Reviews and revises diagnoses, expected outcomes, and the plan of care based on the data collected and the consensus of the health care team.

F. Documents the findings of the evaluation process and the revised plan of care in the medical record.

STANDARDS OF PROFESSIONAL PERFORMANCE: PEDIATRIC ONCOLOGY CLINICAL NURSE

Standard I. Quality of Care

The pediatric oncology nurse participates in activities that improve the quality and effectiveness of nursing care.

Rationale

The pediatric oncology nurse delivers expert, scientifically based care in a health care environment that is continually changing due to technological and scientific advances in basic and behavioral sciences and information systems. New information must be integrated into current practice and continually evaluated.

Measurement Criteria

The pediatric oncology nurse:

A. Participates in quality assessment and improvement activities as appropriate to the nurse's education and position, which may include:

1. Identifying issues in patient care and care delivery systems.

2. Identifying, collecting, and analyzing data to measure and monitor the effectiveness and outcomes of care.

3. Integrating results of quality assessment and improvement activities into practice.

4. Developing policies and procedures that measure compliance and improve quality of care.

B. Improves quality of care and advances nursing practice throughout the work setting and the community.

C. Contributes to systematic knowledge development and research related to the child's and the family's response to care.

D. Integrates results of scientific inquiry and quality assessment and improvement activities into all areas of nursing practice as appropriate.

E. Applies knowledge to improve nursing practice, care delivery systems, and patient care outcomes.

Standard II. Performance Appraisal

The pediatric oncology nurse evaluates one's own nursing practice in relation to professional practice standards and relevant statutes and regulations.

Rationale

The pediatric oncology nurse delivers expert, scientifically based care to children and families in accordance with nursing practice standards established by the profession. Performance appraisal includes self-evaluation and input from peers in accordance with current professional nursing standards.

Measurement Criteria

The pediatric oncology nurse:

A. Demonstrates competency in areas relevant to pediatric oncology nursing practice.

B. Practices according to the knowledge of current professional practice standards, laws, and regulations.

C. Contributes to systematic knowledge development and research by integrating scientific inquiry into areas of practice and decision-making.

D. Engages in regular performance appraisal of one's own clinical practice and role performance, identifying areas of strength and areas for further development and improvement.

E. Demonstrates understanding of a therapeutic nurse-patient relationship and seeks regular constructive feedback regarding individual practice and role performance.

F. Participates in peer performance appraisal activities when possible.

Standard III. Education

The pediatric oncology nurse demonstrates competency in pediatric oncology nursing practice and maintains current knowledge gained from publications, research findings, and professional activities.

Rationale

The rapid expansion of knowledge pertaining to basic and behavioral sciences, technology, and information systems requires an ongoing commitment to scientific inquiry and learning.

Measurement Criteria

The pediatric oncology nurse:

    A. Participates in ongoing educational activities to expand knowledge, enhance role performance, and increase knowledge of professional issues.

    B. Seeks opportunities to obtain knowledge and experiences necessary to develop and maintain clinical skills.

    C. Seeks to obtain certification per eligibility criteria, to demonstrate continued professional development that reflects practice, experience, and current knowledge in pediatric cancer care.

    D. Maintains and updates knowledge of political, cultural, spiritual, social, health care, and ethical issues related to oncology care and practice setting.

    E. Acknowledges and utilizes colleagues as resources and pursues diverse avenues to enhance knowledge and performance.

Standard IV. Collegiality

The pediatric oncology nurse interacts with and contributes to the professional development of peers, colleagues, and others.

Rationale

The pediatric oncology nurse provides leadership in the professional development of other nurses and health care professionals, demonstrating awareness of learning needs and supporting professional development by acting as a preceptor and mentor.

Measurement Criteria

The pediatric oncology nurse:

A. Works collaboratively and functions as an effective member of the health care team, promoting an environment conducive to collaboration, contribution, and professional communication.

B. Facilitates professional growth of self and others by acting as a preceptor and mentor for new staff and students.

C. Assists colleagues and students in the development of therapeutic relationships with children and families.

D. Participates in peer performance appraisal that is constructive and reflective of oncology nursing practice and professional development.

E. Collaborates with colleagues in conducting research and preparing reports, publications, and presentations.

F. Provides leadership that improves the quality of care and advances nursing practice throughout the work setting and the community.

G. Promotes peer and public awareness of the scope of current nursing practice.

H. Contributes to an environment conducive to clinical education of nursing students and other health care professionals as appropriate.

I. Recognizes and respects colleagues and their contributions.

Standard V. Ethics

The pediatric oncology nurse respects the rights of all children and families and makes decisions and designs interventions that are in agreement with ethical principles.

Rationale

Technological advances and scarce resources in health care have created an environment in which ethical issues frequently arise. The pediatric oncology nurse should advocate for the rights of children with cancer and identify and help to resolve ethical conflicts.

Measurement Criteria

The pediatric oncology nurse:

A. Understands and applies the basic ethical principles of autonomy (right to self-determination), beneficence (do what is in the best interest of the patient), nonmaleficence (do minimal harm), justice, and veracity (truth telling).

B. Examines one's own personal beliefs relating to autonomy, rights of a minor, quality of life, death, suffering, truth telling, equality, and access to care.

C. Identifies available resources when formulating ethical decisions.

D. Maintains confidentiality.

E. Provides quality care to all children, irrespective of race, culture, educational background, religious beliefs, socioeconomic status, or ability to pay.

F. Acts as a patient advocate and assists children and families in developing skills so they can advocate for themselves.

G. Identifies ethical conflicts and seeks to resolve them through multidisciplinary team discussions, including the child and family as appropriate.

H. Addresses advance directives with young adults 18 years of age and older.

I. Seeks to include minors in decision-making as appropriate.

J. Ensures that all children and families receive truthful information regarding diagnosis and treatment.

Standard VI. Collaboration

The pediatric oncology nurse collaborates with children, families, and multidisciplinary team members in providing care.

Rationale

The complexity and intensity of oncology care requires coordinated, ongoing interaction among the child, parents, family members, and the multidisciplinary team. Through the collaborative process, health care providers use their diverse abilities to assess, plan, implement, and evaluate care.

Measurement Criteria

The pediatric oncology nurse:

A. Establishes rapport and supportive ongoing relationships with children, parents, and families.

B. Collaborates with the child, family, and other health care providers in the formulation of goals and the plan of care.

C. Identifies appropriate community resources to promote continuity of care and collaborates with managed care/insurance companies for home care and hospice services.

D. Makes referrals as appropriate.

E. Develops relationships with colleagues that facilitate the mutual involvement in planning and evaluating care.

F. Fosters and promotes an environment that facilitates professional communication and collaboration between oneself and colleagues.

Standard VII. Research

The pediatric oncology nurse contributes to evidence-based nursing through participation in, review of, and application of research.

Rationale

Pediatric oncology nurses contribute to systematic knowledge development and research by integrating scientific inquiry into all areas of practice and decision-making. Knowledge gained from research, quality assessment and improvement activities, publications, and professional activities is utilized to advance clinical care and nursing practice.

Measurement Criteria

The pediatric oncology nurse:

A. Critiques research for application to practice.

B. Applies research findings in the development of policies, procedures, and practice guidelines.

C. Complies with clinical protocol requirements regarding eligibility criteria, treatment regimens, and appropriate specimen and data collection when clinically responsible for children enrolled in research protocols.

D. Participates in the protection of human subjects by ensuring informed consent is obtained prior to initiating treatment.

E. Participates in research activities appropriate to the nurse's education and practice setting.

F. Identifies clinical problems suitable for scientific inquiry, research, and/or quality assessment.

G. Integrates research findings into practice when applicable.

Standard VIII. Resource Utilization

The pediatric oncology nurse effectively manages the environment of care, considering factors related to safety, effectiveness, and cost in planning and delivering care.

Rationale

The pediatric oncology nurse delivers care that is safe and effective, and that utilizes resources efficiently. Clinical and administrative decisions consider available resources and desired outcomes of care, and reflect the ability to prioritize actions and utilize colleagues to achieve desired patient outcomes.

Measurement Criteria

The pediatric oncology nurse:

A. Evaluates factors related to safety, effectiveness, availability, and cost when two or more practice options would result in the same expected outcome.

B. Discusses benefits and cost of treatment when exploring options with the family and members of the health care team as appropriate.

C. Assists the child and family to secure appropriate services and financial resources to address health-related needs.

D. Assists the child and family in becoming informed consumers about the cost, risks, and benefits of treatment and care.

E. Delegates responsibilities for the performance of selected patient care activities as defined by the state nurse practice acts and according to the knowledge and skills of the caregiver.

F. Manages the environment of nursing care by identifying resources necessary to achieve desired outcomes.

G. Makes clinical and management decisions that reflect the ability to prioritize actions and utilize colleagues in achieving desired outcomes.

H. Makes clinical and management decisions that consider available resources as well as desired outcomes of practice.

I. Participates in ongoing evaluation of resource utilization.

ADVANCED PRACTICE NURSING

The advanced practice nurse (APN) must comply with all the standards of care and professional performance described for the clinical nurse. In addition, the APN must blend the important functions of the oncology and pediatric APN. These standards incorporate key aspects of previously published standards from organizations such as the American Nurses Association (ANA 1996, 1998), the Society of Pediatric Nurses (Deatrick et al. 1998), and the Oncology Nursing Society (Lester, Glass, and Owen 1997).

The standards of care describe the competent behaviors of the APN in pediatric oncology. These standards address assessment, diagnosis, outcome identification, planning, implementation, and evaluation. The APN is expected to participate in professional role activities applicable to one's educational level, position, and practice setting. Federal laws and state boards of nursing regulate advanced practice nursing. The APN must be cognizant of relevant legislation regarding advanced practice nursing and practice within the scope of the law for the particular state of residence/practice. The standards of professional performance will address the following areas: quality of care, self-evaluation, education, leadership, ethics, interdisciplinary process, and research.

The APN possesses self-direction in the development and maintenance of competency in practice and enhancement of career goals. This should include membership and participation in professional organizations such as the Association of Pediatric Oncology Nurses, American Nurses Association, Oncology Nursing Society, Society of Pediatric Nurses, and National Association of Pediatric Nurse Associates and Practitioners. Relevant certification in the areas of pediatrics, pediatric oncology, and/or oncology is expected, along with appropriate continuing education and professional development activities. In addition, the APN is expected to be a role model for clinical nurses and other health professionals.

STANDARDS OF CARE:
PEDIATRIC ONCOLOGY ADVANCED PRACTICE NURSE

Standard I. Assessment

The pediatric oncology APN collects data from the child and family, using assessment skills to determine physical, emotional, cultural, and social needs, and the well-being of the child and family.

Rationale

Accurate, holistic assessment of the child and family provides information necessary to formulate the most comprehensive plan of care.

Measurement Criteria

The pediatric oncology APN:

A. Collects information in a manner determined by the condition of the child at the time of the assessment including history and physical examination.

B. Assesses the following areas of existing and potential needs: physical care, growth and development, psychosocial care, education, palliative care, long-term survival, and prevention and early detection.

C. Assesses the child and family throughout treatment, adding and revising data as necessary.

D. Orders diagnostic tests and procedures and interprets clinical data from laboratory values and diagnostic imaging, as well as information from other nurses and consultants involved in the child's care.

E. Utilizes critical thinking in data collection and synthesis of information from multiple sources, such as current nursing and medical literature, conference presentations, and information and statistics from clinical trials.

F. Communicates assessment findings and recommendations to the child, in a developmentally appropriate manner, to the family, and to members of the healthcare team

G. Documents assessment findings clearly in the medical record.

Standard II. Diagnosis

The pediatric oncology APN systematically analyzes the assessment data to identify actual and potential diagnoses.

Rationale

Identifying diagnoses and potential problem areas allows the focus of care to be directed toward appropriate interventions.

Measurement Criteria

The pediatric oncology APN:

   A. Develops diagnoses from assessment data, physical examination, and laboratory and diagnostic test results, using advanced clinical skills.

   B. Ensures that the diagnoses include the seven priority areas of pediatric oncology nursing: physical care, growth and development, psychosocial care, education, palliative care, long-term survival, and prevention and early detection.

   C. Develops differential diagnoses and validates them with the child and family, and with members of the health care team.

   D. Prioritizes diagnoses and resultant actions according to the child's condition and most acute needs at the time of assessment.

   E. Documents diagnoses in a clear, concise, prioritized manner in the medical record.

Standard III. Outcome Identification

The pediatric oncology APN identifies expected outcomes based on the assessment and diagnoses of the child and family in collaboration with the multidisciplinary team when appropriate.

Rationale

The development of expected outcomes focuses nursing care on the specific goals that will help the child and family return to optimal health or experience a peaceful death.

The pediatric oncology APN:

A. Develops outcomes for each diagnosis, taking into consideration the family, age of the child, and psychosocial and cultural background.

B. Includes the following areas in defining outcomes: physical care, growth and development, psychosocial care, education, palliative care, long-term survival, and prevention and early detection.

C. Considers financial and emotional burden to family when establishing desired outcomes, and provides optimal care in the most effective way.

D. Utilizes current research and advanced clinical knowledge in defining realistic, measurable outcomes.

E. Modifies and updates outcomes continually according to changes in the child's condition.

F. Ensures that outcomes are congruent with the wishes of the child and family.

G. Documents the outcomes in the medical record.

Standard IV. Planning

The pediatric oncology APN formulates and implements a plan of treatment and interventions based on the diagnoses to achieve the desired outcomes.

Rationale

A holistic, prioritized plan of care specifies the interventions necessary for obtaining the desired results for the child and family.

Measurement Criteria

The pediatric oncology APN:

A. Prescribes interventions and makes recommendations based on advanced clinical knowledge and current research findings.

B. Ensures that the plan of care includes education of the family about potential acute side effects and late effects of the interventions, and the plan to help minimize these effects whenever possible.

C. Ensures that interventions are also focused on health promotion, restoration, and maintenance.

D. Collaborates with the child, family, and other members of the health care team to develop the plan.

E. Documents the plan of care clearly and concisely in the medical record.

Standard V. Implementation

The pediatric oncology APN utilizes the various components of one's role (case management, consultation, health promotion, education, prescriptive authority, referral, and research) to implement the plan of care.

Rationale

Implementation of the plan of care should lead to the attainment of the expected outcomes for the child and family.

Measurement Criteria

The pediatric oncology APN

A. Prescribes interventions based on current research and advanced clinical knowledge.

B. Prescribes and implements interventions that are within the scope of practice of the APN.

C. Involves the child and family in the implementation of the plan of care as much as possible, taking into consideration their comfort level.

D. Documents interventions and the child's response in the medical record.

Standard Va. Case Management/Coordination of Care

The pediatric oncology APN provides comprehensive clinical co-ordination of care throughout the relationship with the child and family.

Rationale

Case management and coordination of care are cost-effective and provide more comprehensive quality care for the child and family.

Measurement Criteria

The pediatric oncology APN:

A. Coordinates care of the child with cancer along the continuum of health and illness, and in varied settings, including the hospital, ambulatory/multidisciplinary clinics, home, and hospice, as appropriate.

B. Utilizes resource-management techniques to provide the most cost- effective high-quality care.

C. Communicates with the family to assess if all of their needs and the needs of the child are being met.

D. Helps to implement and follow clinical pathways/guidelines that are developed for each diagnosis.

E. Identifies, measures, and analyzes outcomes as indicated for each child and family.

F. Documents case management in the medical record.

Standard Vb. Consultation

The pediatric oncology APN provides consultation to members of the health care team, child, family, and community to influence changes in health care.

Rationale

The APN provides consultation for health issues or problems by drawing on experience and knowledge in pediatric oncology nursing. This expertise enables the APN to offer recommendations for interventions or changes that would improve care for a particular child or for a larger population in general.

Measurement Criteria

The pediatric oncology APN:

A. Provides information and serves as a resource person for children and families, other health care providers, and the community in areas of children's health and pediatric cancer, which may include teaching about clinical trial protocols, palliative care strategies, and survivorship issues.

B. Communicates at a level that is understandable to those without a healthcare background.

C. Maintains up-to-date knowledge by reviewing current literature and attending conferences.

D. Networks with other healthcare professionals to share knowledge and resources to provide the best care available.

E. Consults with nursing administration to provide education and clinical supervision for clinical nurses.

F. Collaborates with nursing administration to identify competency-based skills needed to evaluate staff performance.

Standard Vc. Health Promotion, Health Maintenance, and Health Teaching

The pediatric oncology APN uses complex strategies and interventions to promote and maintain a return to health, with minimal complications and late effects of therapy. The APN also provides teaching regarding pediatric and oncology health concerns to children, their families, and the community.

Rationale

The health continuum covers the spectrum of health maintenance from acute or chronic illness to recovery or death. The APN provides guidance and education throughout the continuum.

Measurement Criteria

The pediatric oncology APN:

A. Assesses the need for and provides interventions and education in the areas of health promotion, recovery, and health maintenance.

B. Provides consultation based on knowledge of epidemiologic and cultural variables.

C. Provides education based on the educational and developmental level of the individual or audience.

D. Collaborates with nursing administration and other colleagues to develop educational programs for children and families.

Standard Vd. Prescriptive Authority and Treatment

The pediatric oncology APN uses prescriptive authority in accordance with state and federal regulations in prescribing or furnishing medications and treatments, and in performing procedures essential to the diagnosis and treatment of children with cancer.

Rationale

Advanced practice nursing is regulated by state boards of nursing and by the clinical privileges granted within each institution.

Measurement Criteria

The pediatric oncology APN:

A. Prescribes or administers specific medications based on knowledge of pharmacology, physiology, and current research findings in cancer care.

B. Prescribes or administers specific medications with the intent to treat illness, improve functional health status, or provide preventive care.

C. Adheres to rules and regulations related to the dispensing of medications and treatments.

D. Informs the child and family about potential side effects and/or late effects of medications and treatments given.

E. Provides cost information and facts about alternative therapies.

F. Monitors for expected and potential effects of medications and has appropriate interventions in place to treat or minimize these effects.

G. Competently performs procedures such as bone marrow aspirates, biopsies, and lumbar punctures as appropriate to the setting and institutional collaborative practice arrangements.

Standard Ve. Referral

The pediatric oncology APN, in consultation with the primary oncologist as appropriate, makes referrals based on the need for additional resources or a consultation by a specialist.

Rationale

Referral should be made for any need that is outside the APN's scope of practice or area of expertise.

Measurement Criteria

The pediatric oncology APN:

A. Recognizes one's own scope of practice and consults with the primary oncologist as needed.

B. Makes referrals that are most cost-effective and beneficial to the child, working within the child's health care coverage whenever possible.

C. Communicates with the specialist to provide continuity of care.

D. Remains available to the specialist and follows up on recommendations.

Standard VI. Evaluation

The pediatric oncology APN evaluates the response to the plan and interventions, and monitors the progress toward achievement of expected outcomes.

Rationale

Evaluation allows for determination of reaching goals, and if goals are not met, for reassessing and redefining plan and goals.

Measurement Criteria

The pediatric oncology APN:

    A. Develops and maintains a systematic and effective evaluation process.

    B. Involves other members of the health care team and the child and family in the evaluation process.

    C. Evaluates the child's response to interventions and current health status.

    D. Bases evaluation on advanced nursing knowledge and current research findings.

    E. Revises plan and interventions as necessary.

    F. Documents evaluation results and revised plan or resolution in the medical record.

STANDARDS OF PROFESSIONAL PERFORMANCE: PEDIATRIC ONCOLOGY ADVANCED PRACTICE NURSE

Standard I. Quality of Care

The pediatric oncology APN systematically develops criteria for and evaluates the quality of care for clinical outcomes and the effectiveness of clinical and advanced pediatric oncology nursing practice.

Rationale

The APN delivers expert care in a health care environment that is continually changing due to technological and scientific advances in basic and behavioral sciences and information systems. The APN is expected to be a leader in the development of patient care standards and the evaluation of outcomes.

Measurement Criteria

The pediatric oncology APN:

A. Develops and monitors standards of care to improve the care of the child with cancer and family in collaboration with other health care team members.

B. Analyzes outcome data from the literature and quality improvement processes to identify necessary changes that will improve pediatric oncology care throughout the health care system.

C. Involves children and families in the analysis of quality improvement activities.

D. Collaborates with the health care team to coordinate quality of care activities and to formulate comprehensive plans to provide high-quality and cost-effective care.

Standard II. Self-Evaluation

The pediatric oncology APN evaluates one's own clinical practice to provide competent care and is accountable to the public and the profession.

The APN functions with a high degree of independence and must assume responsibility for self-evaluation by soliciting input from superiors, peers, and colleagues.

Measurement Criteria

The pediatric oncology APN:

    A. Evaluates one's own advanced nursing practice in regard to institutional, state, and federal laws and regulations as well as child and family outcomes.

    B. Seeks feedback from peers, colleagues, health care team members, and child/family regarding practice and performance.

    C. Identifies personal strengths and weaknesses and independently seeks opportunities to meet educational and other performance goals.

    D. Communicates areas of concern regarding performance of peers and other health care professionals in a professional and ethical manner.

Standard III. Education

The pediatric oncology APN acquires and maintains current knowledge and skills in the area of pediatric oncology nursing and related disciplines as appropriate.

Rationale

The rapid expansion of knowledge pertaining to basic and behavioral sciences, technology, and information systems requires ongoing commitment to scientific inquiry and learning.

Measurement Criteria

The pediatric oncology APN:

    A. Seeks out and participates in educational opportunities to expand clinical knowledge, perform research, enhance role performance, and increase knowledge of professional issues.

B. Maintains specialized education, certification, and licensure requirements according to institutional, state, and federal laws and regulations.

Standard IV. Leadership

The APN serves as a leader, role model, and mentor for the professional development of peers, colleagues, staff, and students.

Rationale

The APN is considered the nursing clinical expert and must demonstrate leadership skills to promote nursing care delivered to children and families as well as the profession of pediatric oncology nursing.

Measurement Criteria

The pediatric oncology APN:

A. Contributes to the professional development and education of others regarding pediatric oncology nursing.

B. Participates in professional and specialty nursing organizations, as well as advocacy and service organizations related to pediatric oncology.

C. Presents and publishes in the area of pediatric oncology.

D. Proactively fosters a learning environment by serving as a role model, mentor, preceptor, and facilitator of learning for pediatric oncology nurses and APNs.

E. Serves as a liaison to other professional, advocacy, and legislative organizations to influence advanced practice nursing and the care of children with cancer and their families.

Standard V. Ethics

The APN respects the rights of all children and families and makes decisions and designs interventions that are in agreement with ethical principles.

Rationale

Technological advances and scarce resources have created an environment in which ethical issues frequently arise. The APN is a clinical professional leader who must advocate for patient and family rights and assist others in resolving conflicts.

Measurement Criteria

The pediatric oncology APN:

A. Instructs others and models ethical nursing practice by applying the basic ethical principles autonomy, beneficence, nonmaleficence, justice and veracity.

B. Examines one's own views and helps others to assess personal beliefs about autonomy, rights of minors, quality of life, death, suffering, truth telling, equality, and access to care.

C. Educates children and families about informed decision-making.

D. Maintains confidentiality.

E. Ensures that Institutional Review Board (IRB) regulations are followed in clinical trials and developmentally appropriate child assent is obtained as indicated.

F. Identifies ethical conflicts and seeks to resolve them through multidisciplinary team discussions, including the child and family as appropriate.

G. Reviews institutional policies and procedures that relate to biomedical or organizational ethics as appropriate.

H. Provides quality care to all children, irrespective of race, educational background, socioeconomic status, or ability to pay.

I. Addresses advance directives with young adults 18 years of age and older.

J. Ensures that all children and families receive truthful information regarding diagnosis and treatment.

Standard VI. Interdisciplinary Process

The APN promotes and collaborates with the multidisciplinary team to care for the child and family.

Rationale

The complexity of pediatric oncology care requires coordinated, ongoing interaction among the members of the multidisciplinary team. Through collaborative practice, the APN works with other team members to care for the child and family.

Measurement Criteria

The pediatric oncology APN:

   A.   Collaborates with multidisciplinary health care team members in providing care.

   B.   Collaborates within the Children's Oncology Group and other research groups to develop research and clinical trials for treatment of the child with cancer.

   C.   Consults with other disciplines to improve care.

   D.   Collaborates with other disciplines and members of the health care team regarding continuity of care, rehabilitation, home care, symptom management, palliative care, and hospice care.

   E.   Works collaboratively with parents to ensure optimal care is provided to children with cancer.

Standard VII. Research

The APN strives to maintain an evidence-based practice and contributes to nursing knowledge through the incorporation of research activities into practice.

Rationale

Through advanced education and practice, the APN is in a position to contribute significantly to the identification of pertinent questions for research in pediatric oncology nursing. The APN may, as an individual or in collaboration with others, design and conduct studies to answer important questions that impact the care of the child and family.

Measurement Criteria

The pediatric oncology APN:

A. Promotes evidence-based practice in all areas of pediatric oncology nursing.

B. Examines and evaluates research.

C. Examines and evaluates practice in regard to current research findings.

D. Develops testable hypotheses and research proposals when indicated.

E. Serves as resource to staff nurses regarding the research process and research-based nursing practice.

F. Collaborates with others to develop research.

G. Participates in Children's Oncology Group or other clinical trials research through the development, implementation, and evaluation of pediatric clinical trials.

H. Disseminates research findings through practice, education, or consultation.

I. Ensures the protection of research subjects.

REFERENCES

ANA (American Nurses Association) 2000. *Recognition of a Specialty, Approval of Scope Statements and Acknowledgment of Nursing Practice Standards*. Washington, DC: American Nurses Association.

————. 1998. *Standards of Clinical Nursing Practice*. 2d edition. Washington, DC: American Nurses Association.

————. 1996. *Scope and Standards of Advanced Practice Registered Nursing*. Washington, DC: American Nurses Association.

————. 1985. *Code for Nurses with Interpretive Statements*. Washington, DC: American Nurses Association.

APON (Association of Pediatric Oncology Nurses) 2000. *Scope of Practice and Outcome Standard of Practice for Pediatric Oncology Nurses*. Glenville, Illinois: Association of Pediatric Oncology Nurses.

————. 1995. *Job Analysis*. Glenville, Illinois: Association Management Center.

Bartolone, C., K. Carroll, J. Deatrick, L. Bakken, L. Lewandowski, and L. Linden. 1996. *Statement on the Scope and Standards of Pediatric Clinical Nursing Practice*. Society of Pediatric Nurses and American Nurses Association.

Bleyer, A., H. Tejeda, S. Murphy, L. Robison, J. Ross, B. Bollecok, F. Severson, O. Brawley, M. Smith, and R. Ungerleider. 1997. National cancer clinical trials: children have equal access; adolescents do not. *Journal of Adolescent Health* 21:366-373.

Brant, J. M., R. R. Iwamoto, K. A. Rumsey, and B. L. Young Summers. 1996. *Statement on the Scope and Standards of Oncology Nursing Practice*. Washington, DC: Oncology Nursing Society and American Nurses Association.

Bru, G., J. Chiavello, K. Hegranes, C. Walker, L. Wofford, P. Wright, and G. Foley. 1987. *Scope of Practice and Outcome Standards of Practice for Pediatric Oncology Nursing*. Richmond, Virginia: Association of Pediatric Oncology Nurses.

Deatrick, J., C. Bartolone, M. Broome, M. Curley, B. Durand, L. Linden, M. Miles, M. Perkins, M. Savedra, and J. Verger. 1998. *Statement on the Scope and Standards of Advanced Practice Pediatric Nursing.* Unpublished manuscript available upon request. Pensacola, Florida: Society of Pediatric Nurses.

Hockenberry-Eaton, M (Ed.). 1998. *Essentials of Pediatric Oncology Nursing: A Core Curriculum.* Glenville, Illinois: Association of Pediatric Oncology Nurses.

Lester, J., E. Glass, and E. Owen. 1997. *Statement on the Scope and Standards of Advanced Practice in Oncology Nursing.* Pittsburgh: Oncology Nursing Press.